Common Misconceptions about Yoga

Many people hold misconceptions about yoga that can deter them from exploring its numerous benefits. One prevalent belief is that yoga is only for the young and flexible. This notion can discourage seniors, athletes, and individuals with varying levels of fitness from participating in yoga. In reality, yoga is accessible to everyone, regardless of age or physical ability. Gentle flow practices are specifically designed to accommodate seniors and those recovering from injuries, allowing for modifications and variations that make yoga a safe and beneficial practice for all.

Another common misconception is that yoga is solely a physical exercise focused on flexibility and strength. While these aspects are indeed important, yoga encompasses much more than just physical postures. It includes mental and emotional dimensions, promoting mindfulness and relaxation. This holistic approach allows individuals to enhance their mental health, reduce stress, and cultivate a sense of inner peace. For office workers and busy parents, incorporating yoga into their routine can provide essential moments of calm and clarity amidst their hectic lives.

Many believe that yoga requires a significant time commitment to be effective. This misconception can be particularly discouraging for those with tight schedules, including athletes and working professionals. However, yoga can be practiced in short sessions, making it flexible to fit even the busiest lifestyles. Whether through a quick morning routine or a brief evening unwind, even ten minutes of yoga can lead to noticeable improvements in flexibility, balance, and overall well-being.

Some people also assume that yoga is a solitary practice, leading to the false belief that it lacks community support. In truth, yoga can foster a strong sense of community and connection among practitioners. Many studios and classes offer group settings where participants can share their experiences and support one another in their journeys. This social aspect is particularly beneficial for seniors and those seeking mental health benefits, as it encourages social interaction and reduces feelings of isolation.

Lastly, the idea that yoga is only for those seeking weight loss is a misconception that overlooks the diverse purposes of yoga practice. While certain styles, like hot yoga or vigorous flow, can aid in weight management, many forms of yoga focus on relaxation, restorative practices, and injury recovery. This makes yoga an excellent choice for individuals dealing with back pain or those simply looking to enhance their overall quality of life. By dispelling these misconceptions, individuals of all backgrounds can embrace yoga as a powerful tool for personal growth and health.

Chapter 2: The Foundations of Gentle Flow Yoga

Key Principles of Gentle Flow

Gentle Flow yoga is rooted in principles that prioritize safety, comfort, and accessibility, making it an ideal practice for people of all ages and fitness levels. One of the key principles is the focus on mindful movement. This involves cultivating awareness of the body and breath while transitioning between poses. By encouraging practitioners to move slowly and deliberately, Gentle Flow fosters a deeper connection to the body, which is particularly beneficial for seniors and individuals recovering from injuries. This mindful approach not only enhances flexibility and balance but also supports mental clarity and emotional well-being.

Another essential principle of Gentle Flow is the emphasis on alignment and body awareness. Proper alignment is critical in preventing injuries, especially for seniors and those who may have pre-existing conditions. Gentle Flow encourages modifications and the use of props, such as blocks and straps, to ensure that each practitioner can find the correct alignment in their poses. This principle of inclusivity allows everyone, from office workers to athletes, to adapt their practice to suit their individual needs, enhancing their physical capabilities while minimizing strain.

Breath is a fundamental aspect of Gentle Flow. Integrating breath with movement creates a harmonious flow that promotes relaxation and reduces stress. This principle is especially relevant for individuals seeking mental health benefits through yoga. By focusing on the breath, practitioners can cultivate a calming presence that enhances mindfulness and encourages a meditative state. This deep breathing practice not only supports overall mental wellness but can also aid in physical recovery, making it a beneficial practice for athletes and those dealing with chronic pain or recovery from injuries.

The principle of pacing is vital in Gentle Flow, allowing practitioners to progress at their own speed. This aspect is crucial for seniors and anyone new to yoga, as it helps prevent overwhelm and encourages a steady, sustainable practice. Gentle Flow recognizes that each individual's journey is unique, and by allowing space for personal growth, it fosters a supportive environment where practitioners can build confidence in their abilities. This principle also aids in weight management and physical conditioning, as the gentle pacing encourages consistency without the risk of burnout.

Lastly, the incorporation of restorative elements is a hallmark of Gentle Flow. This principle recognizes the importance of rest and recovery in any exercise routine. Gentle Flow includes longer-held poses and restorative sequences that allow the body to release tension and rejuvenate. This is particularly beneficial for seniors and those experiencing back pain, as it promotes healing and relaxation. The restorative aspect also serves to enhance the mindfulness experience, allowing practitioners to fully immerse themselves in the present moment, thus reaping the full mental and physical benefits of their yoga practice.

Chapter 1: Introduction to Yoga for Seniors

Understanding the Importance of Yoga in Later Life

Understanding the importance of yoga in later life extends beyond the physical benefits, touching upon mental, emotional, and social well-being. As individuals age, they often experience a decline in flexibility, strength, and balance, which can lead to an increased risk of injury and a decrease in overall quality of life. Incorporating yoga into a daily routine can counteract these changes, enhancing mobility and stability. Gentle flow yoga, specifically tailored for seniors, emphasizes safe movements that promote joint health and muscle tone, providing a foundation for improved physical function.

Yoga also plays a crucial role in mental health, particularly for seniors. Engaging in yoga practices can alleviate symptoms of anxiety and depression, often prevalent in older adults. The mindfulness aspect of yoga encourages practitioners to focus on the present moment, fostering a sense of peace and reducing stress. Regular yoga sessions can enhance cognitive function, helping to maintain clarity and focus as one ages. This mental engagement is vital for overall well-being, as it keeps the mind active and sharp.

Social interaction is another significant benefit of practicing yoga, especially in later life. Group classes create a community environment where seniors can connect with others, reducing feelings of isolation and loneliness. The shared experience of yoga fosters camaraderie and support among participants, promoting a sense of belonging. This social engagement is essential for emotional health, as it encourages individuals to develop friendships and support systems, which are vital as they navigate the challenges of aging.

Restorative yoga is particularly beneficial for seniors, focusing on relaxation and gentle stretches that can be adapted to individual needs. This form of yoga allows for deep relaxation and encourages the body to heal itself, making it an excellent option for those dealing with chronic pain or limited mobility. By incorporating restorative practices into their routine, seniors can experience improved sleep, reduced tension, and enhanced overall well-being.

Lastly, the importance of yoga in later life extends to its ability to promote healthy lifestyle choices. Regular practice can motivate seniors to engage in other physical activities, maintain a healthy diet, and prioritize self-care. This holistic approach not only addresses physical limitations but also encourages a balanced lifestyle that supports longevity and vitality. By embracing yoga, seniors can enhance their quality of life, fostering resilience and adaptability as they navigate the later stages of their journey.

Benefits of Yoga for Seniors

Yoga offers a multitude of benefits for seniors, enhancing both physical and mental well-being. As individuals age, maintaining flexibility and balance becomes increasingly crucial to prevent falls and injuries. Gentle yoga practices focus on slow, deliberate movements that promote joint mobility and muscular strength. By incorporating poses specifically designed for seniors, such as seated stretches and gentle twists, practitioners can improve their range of motion and overall physical resilience. This gradual approach allows seniors to engage in physical activity without the risk of strain, making yoga an accessible form of exercise for all fitness levels.

In addition to physical benefits, yoga serves as an effective tool for mental health among seniors. The practice encourages mindfulness through breath awareness and focused attention, helping to reduce stress and anxiety. Engaging in regular yoga sessions can foster a sense of calm and tranquility, which is particularly beneficial for seniors who may experience loneliness or depression. By cultivating a mindful approach to life, seniors can enhance their emotional well-being, leading to improved mood and a greater sense of connection with themselves and others.

Yoga also plays a significant role in promoting better sleep quality for seniors. Many older adults struggle with sleep disturbances due to various factors, including pain and anxiety. Restorative yoga practices, which involve gentle stretches and relaxation techniques, can help quiet the mind and prepare the body for restful sleep. By incorporating restorative poses into their routine, seniors can alleviate tension, calm their nervous system, and create a conducive environment for deeper, more restorative sleep patterns. This improvement in sleep quality can further contribute to their overall health and vitality.

Another noteworthy benefit of yoga for seniors is its potential for pain relief, particularly concerning back pain, which is a common complaint in this age group. Specific yoga poses can strengthen the core muscles that support the spine, reducing pressure and discomfort. Additionally, yoga promotes flexibility in the back and hips, which can alleviate stiffness and improve posture. Regular practice not only aids in managing existing pain but can also prevent future discomfort by encouraging proper alignment and movement patterns.

Lastly, yoga fosters a sense of community and social interaction among seniors, which is essential for maintaining a healthy lifestyle. Group yoga classes provide opportunities for seniors to connect with others, share experiences, and support one another in their wellness journeys. This social component is vital for combating feelings of isolation and enhancing overall quality of life. By participating in yoga, seniors can build friendships, find a sense of belonging, and engage in meaningful activities that contribute to their physical and emotional health.

Basic Poses for Flexibility and Balance

Flexibility and balance are essential components of physical health, particularly as we age or engage in various physical activities. Incorporating basic yoga poses into your routine can significantly enhance these attributes, providing benefits not only for seniors but for athletes, office workers, and individuals from all walks of life. Yoga promotes a mindful connection between body and mind, making it a valuable practice for promoting overall well-being. This subchapter will explore several foundational poses that can be easily integrated into daily routines to improve flexibility and balance.

The Mountain Pose, or Tadasana, serves as a fundamental starting point for many yoga practices. Standing tall with feet together, grounding through the feet while engaging the thighs and lifting the chest offers a strong foundation for balance. This pose encourages proper posture and alignment while instilling a sense of stability. It is particularly beneficial for seniors, as it strengthens the legs and core, reducing the risk of falls. For office workers and athletes, this pose also helps to counteract the effects of prolonged sitting and enhances awareness of body alignment.

The Tree Pose, or Vrksasana, is another excellent pose for improving balance and flexibility. This pose involves standing on one leg while placing the sole of the opposite foot on the inner thigh or calf of the standing leg. The arms can be raised overhead or positioned in front of the heart. The Tree Pose challenges stability and encourages concentration, making it effective for mental clarity as well. It is especially useful for athletes seeking to improve their balance during dynamic activities, as well as seniors looking to build strength in the legs and core while enhancing their overall equilibrium.

Incorporating seated poses, such as the Seated Forward Bend (Paschimottanasana), can greatly increase flexibility, especially in the hamstrings and lower back. Sitting with legs extended, hinging at the hips to reach forward, allows for a gentle stretch while promoting relaxation. This pose is particularly beneficial for those dealing with back pain or stiffness, as it nurtures a calming effect on the nervous system. Mindfulness plays a key role in this pose, encouraging practitioners to focus on their breath and listen to their bodies, making it suitable for individuals of all ages and fitness levels.

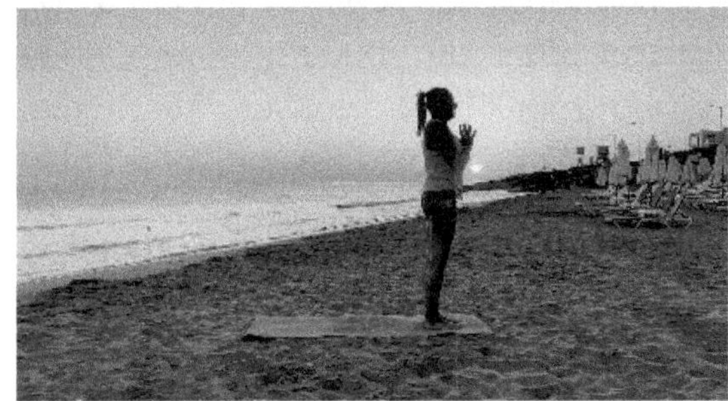

Tadasana (Mountain Pose)

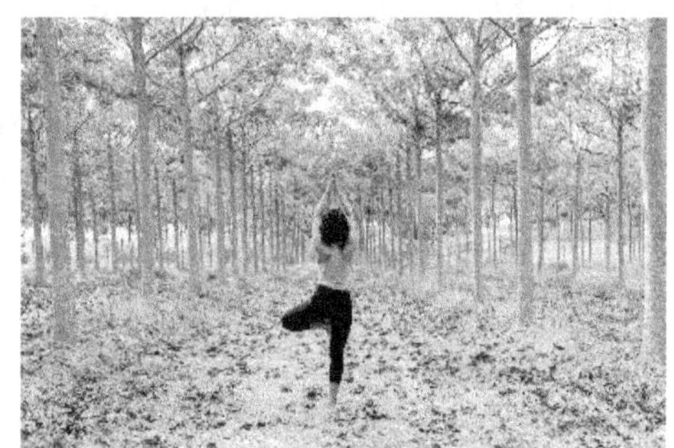

Vrksasana (Tree Pose)

Finally, the Cat-Cow Stretch (Marjaryasana-Bitilasana) is a dynamic pose that fosters flexibility in the spine and promotes balance between movement and stillness. Alternating between arching and rounding the back while on all fours allows for increased mobility in the spine, while also strengthening the core. This stretch is beneficial for office workers and seniors, as it alleviates tension in the back and promotes better posture. Additionally, the rhythmic nature of this pose encourages mindfulness, making it a great way to connect breath with movement and find a sense of calm amidst a busy day.

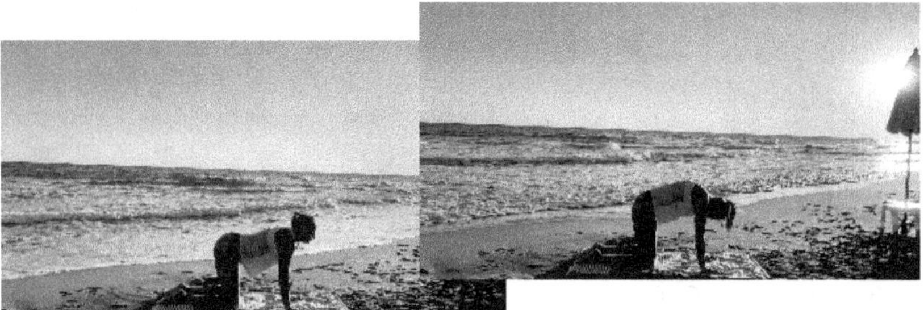

Cat Cow

In conclusion, integrating basic yoga poses into your daily routine can significantly enhance flexibility and balance for individuals of all ages and fitness levels. Through consistent practice of poses such as Mountain Pose, Tree Pose, Seated Forward Bend, and Cat-Cow Stretch, practitioners can build strength, improve posture, and cultivate a deeper sense of awareness. Whether you are a senior seeking to maintain mobility, an athlete aiming for peak performance, or simply someone looking to enhance overall well-being, these foundational poses provide a gentle yet effective pathway to achieving your goals.

Breathing Techniques for Relaxation

Breathing techniques are fundamental tools in yoga that promote relaxation and enhance overall well-being. These practices can be easily integrated into daily routines, making them accessible to everyone, from busy parents and office workers to seniors and athletes. By focusing on the breath, individuals can cultivate a deeper sense of calm, reduce stress, and improve mental clarity. In this subchapter, we will explore various breathing techniques that can be particularly beneficial for enhancing relaxation and promoting mindfulness.

One effective technique is diaphragmatic breathing, which encourages full oxygen exchange and can activate the body's relaxation response. To practice diaphragmatic breathing, begin by finding a comfortable seated or lying position. Place one hand on your chest and the other on your abdomen. Inhale deeply through your nose, allowing your abdomen to rise while keeping your chest relatively still. Exhale slowly through your mouth, feeling your abdomen fall. This technique not only promotes relaxation but also helps to alleviate tension and anxiety, making it suitable for individuals of all ages and backgrounds.

Another popular technique is the 4-7-8 breathing method, which can be particularly beneficial for those struggling with stress or insomnia. This technique involves inhaling through the nose for four counts, holding the breath for seven counts, and exhaling through the mouth for eight counts. Repeat this cycle several times. The 4-7-8 method can effectively calm the nervous system and induce a state of relaxation, making it a valuable tool for athletes looking to enhance their performance or for seniors seeking to improve their mental health and emotional well-being.

Box breathing is another simple yet powerful technique that can be practiced anywhere, making it ideal for office workers or busy parents. This method consists of four equal parts: inhale for four counts, hold for four counts, exhale for four counts, and hold for four counts before inhaling again. Box breathing helps to focus the mind, reduce stress levels, and promote a sense of balance. It can be particularly useful during moments of high stress, helping individuals to regain control and center themselves.

Finally, incorporating breath awareness into yoga practice can enhance relaxation and mindfulness. As practitioners move through gentle flows, focusing on the breath can deepen the connection between mind and body. This approach not only aids in maintaining balance and flexibility but also fosters a sense of presence and tranquility. By integrating these breathing techniques into daily life and yoga practice, individuals can experience improved emotional health, increased relaxation, and a greater sense of overall well-being.

Chapter 3: Enhancing Flexibility

Importance of Flexibility in Aging

Flexibility plays a crucial role in the aging process, impacting not just physical health but also mental well-being. As individuals age, their bodies naturally undergo changes that can lead to decreased flexibility. This can result in a range of issues, including reduced mobility, increased risk of injury, and chronic pain. Maintaining flexibility is essential for seniors, as it promotes better posture and alignment, which can alleviate stress on the joints and spine. Moreover, enhancing flexibility through practices like yoga can significantly improve overall functional capacity, enabling seniors to engage more fully in daily activities.

Incorporating flexibility-enhancing exercises into daily routines is particularly beneficial for seniors. Gentle yoga practices are designed to stretch and strengthen the muscles without straining them. These practices help maintain joint health, improve circulation, and enhance balance, which is vital for preventing falls—one of the leading causes of injury among older adults. By fostering flexibility, seniors can enjoy a greater range of motion, making it easier to perform everyday tasks such as bending down to tie shoes or reaching for objects on high shelves.

For younger individuals, including office workers and athletes, flexibility is equally important. Many desk-bound workers experience tightness in the hips, back, and shoulders due to prolonged periods of sitting. Incorporating flexibility exercises into their routines can counteract these effects, reducing discomfort and enhancing productivity. On the other hand, athletes benefit from improved flexibility by allowing for better performance and reducing the risk of injuries. Yoga can serve as an excellent complement to traditional training, ensuring that muscles remain supple and resilient, which is essential for peak athletic performance.

Mindfulness is another key component of flexibility, particularly as it relates to mental health. Practicing yoga not only stretches the body but also encourages a mindful approach to movement and breath. This mindfulness can help reduce stress and anxiety, contributing to emotional resilience. For seniors, this is especially important as they may face various life transitions that can be challenging. By fostering a flexible mindset through yoga, individuals of all ages can learn to adapt to change more gracefully and maintain a positive outlook on life.

Ultimately, the importance of flexibility in aging cannot be overstated. Whether for seniors looking to maintain independence, office workers aiming to counteract the effects of a sedentary lifestyle, or athletes seeking to enhance their performance, flexibility is a vital aspect of overall health and well-being. Embracing practices such as restorative yoga can promote not only physical flexibility but also mental and emotional adaptability, making it an invaluable tool for people at every stage of life.

Gentle Stretches for Daily Practice

Gentle stretches are an essential part of any daily routine, particularly for those looking to enhance flexibility and balance. These stretches can be easily incorporated into the lives of everyone, from seniors seeking increased mobility to office workers needing a break from prolonged sitting. Gentle stretches not only improve physical flexibility but also promote mental well-being, making them an excellent addition to any practice, whether for athletes or those simply looking to unwind after a long day.

One of the key benefits of gentle stretches is their accessibility. They can be performed anytime and anywhere, requiring no special equipment. Simple movements like neck rolls, shoulder shrugs, and seated forward bends can significantly alleviate tension and discomfort associated with daily tasks. For seniors, these stretches can help maintain joint health and prevent stiffness, while for office workers, they provide a quick way to counteract the negative effects of sitting for extended periods. Incorporating these stretches into your day can lead to improved posture and a greater sense of ease in daily activities.

Incorporating mindfulness into your stretching routine can enhance both physical and mental health. By focusing on your breath and the sensations in your body, you create a meditative experience that encourages relaxation and stress relief. This approach is especially beneficial for individuals dealing with anxiety or mental fatigue. Athletes can also benefit from this mindful aspect, as it helps them stay present and connected to their bodies, improving their overall performance and recovery.

For those managing specific issues like back pain or weight loss, gentle stretches can be tailored to address these concerns. Techniques such as gentle twists and supported backbends can relieve tension in the spine and promote better alignment. Moreover, when combined with a mindful approach, these stretches can enhance body awareness, encouraging healthier habits and movements throughout the day. Consistent practice can lead to gradual improvements, making daily activities more comfortable and enjoyable.

In conclusion, gentle stretches are a versatile and beneficial practice for individuals of all ages and lifestyles. By dedicating just a few minutes each day to these movements, you can enhance your flexibility, improve your balance, and foster a deeper connection with your body and mind. Whether you're a senior looking to maintain mobility, an athlete seeking recovery, or anyone in between, integrating gentle stretches into your daily routine can lead to a healthier, more balanced life.

Incorporating Props for Better Support

Incorporating props into yoga practice can significantly enhance the experience for practitioners of all ages and abilities. Props such as blocks, straps, bolsters, and blankets serve as valuable tools to provide additional support and stability during poses. For seniors, the use of props can help ease the strain on joints and promote safe alignment, allowing for a more comfortable practice. For athletes, props can assist in deepening stretches and improving overall muscle engagement. Understanding how to effectively integrate these tools can lead to a more fulfilling yoga experience, whether for enhancing flexibility, balance, or mental clarity.

Blocks are perhaps the most versatile props available to yogis. They can elevate the ground for poses like forward bends, making them more accessible and reducing the risk of injury. For seniors, blocks can help maintain proper alignment without overexerting. Athletes can use blocks to facilitate deeper stretches in poses like triangle or extended side angle, aiding in muscle recovery and flexibility. By incorporating blocks into your practice, you can modify poses to suit your individual needs while still experiencing the benefits of each posture.

Straps are another essential tool that can aid in both flexibility and alignment. They are particularly useful for individuals who may find certain stretches challenging. For seniors, using a strap can help reach the feet in seated forward bends, enhancing the stretch without straining the back. Athletes can use straps to assist in deepening shoulder stretches or to maintain proper form during challenging poses. By holding onto a strap, practitioners can gradually increase their range of motion over time, promoting better flexibility and reducing the risk of injury.

Bolsters and blankets provide additional support and comfort, making restorative poses more accessible. For seniors, these props can create a sense of security and relaxation, allowing for a deeper engagement with restorative practices that promote mental health and overall well-being. Athletes can benefit from bolsters during recovery sessions, allowing the body to rest and restore while still receiving the benefits of gentle stretches. Incorporating bolsters and blankets into your practice can facilitate a nurturing environment that encourages mindfulness and relaxation, which is crucial for stress management and mental clarity.

Finally, the mindful use of props can enhance the overall yoga experience by fostering a sense of awareness and presence in each pose. Whether you are a parent seeking to balance a busy lifestyle, an office worker looking to alleviate tension, or a senior focusing on maintaining mobility, props can create a supportive environment conducive to personal growth and healing. By embracing the use of props in your yoga practice, you not only enhance flexibility and balance but also cultivate a deeper connection to your body and mind, paving the way for a more enriching and holistic yoga journey.

Chapter 4: Building Balance

Understanding Balance and Stability

Understanding balance and stability is essential for individuals of all ages, particularly for seniors, athletes, and those engaged in daily office activities. Balance refers to the ability to maintain the body's center of mass over its base of support, while stability involves the ability to control this balance in various positions and movements. As we age, our balance can diminish due to physical changes, decreased muscle strength, and reduced coordination. This decline can lead to an increased risk of falls and injuries, making it crucial to incorporate practices that enhance balance and stability into our daily routines.

Yoga serves as a powerful tool for improving balance and stability through its emphasis on mindful movement and body awareness. The practice encourages individuals to engage in various poses that challenge their balance, such as Tree Pose and Warrior III. These poses not only strengthen the muscles involved in maintaining balance but also improve proprioception, which is the body's ability to sense its position in space. By regularly practicing yoga, individuals can develop a stronger foundation, enabling them to perform everyday tasks with greater ease and confidence.

For seniors, maintaining balance and stability is particularly important. As physical capabilities change with age, yoga provides a safe and supportive environment to strengthen core muscles and enhance flexibility. Restorative yoga, with its focus on gentle movements and supportive props, can be especially beneficial for seniors, helping to alleviate pain and increase stability without putting undue stress on the body. This mindful approach to movement encourages seniors to listen to their bodies, fostering a deeper connection and understanding of their physical limits.

Athletes, too, can benefit significantly from a dedicated yoga practice. Balance and stability are critical components of athletic performance, impacting everything from running to weightlifting. Incorporating yoga can help athletes cultivate greater body awareness, refine their techniques, and prevent injuries. Many athletes find that yoga not only improves their physical abilities but also enhances their mental focus, allowing them to perform at their best under competitive conditions. By integrating yoga into their training regimen, athletes can achieve a more well-rounded approach to their physical fitness.

In addition to physical benefits, understanding balance and stability through yoga can greatly enhance mental health. The practice promotes mindfulness, allowing individuals to tune into their breath and body, reducing stress and anxiety. This mental clarity can lead to improved focus and concentration, which are essential for success in both athletic endeavors and everyday life. By prioritizing balance and stability in their yoga practice, individuals across all demographics can cultivate a sense of well-being that extends beyond the mat, enriching their overall quality of life.

Poses to Improve Balance

Incorporating specific yoga poses into your routine can greatly enhance balance, an essential component of physical health for individuals of all ages and fitness levels. Balance is not only crucial for physical stability but also plays a significant role in preventing falls and injuries, particularly among seniors. By practicing poses that challenge your stability, you can build strength in the core and lower body while improving coordination and mental focus. These benefits are valuable for everyone, including office workers who may spend long hours sitting, athletes looking to improve performance, and seniors aiming to maintain their independence.

One effective pose for improving balance is the Tree Pose (Vrksasana). This pose encourages individuals to root one foot firmly into the ground while the other foot rests against the inner thigh or calf of the standing leg. By focusing on a fixed point in front of you, the Tree Pose not only strengthens the legs but also enhances concentration and mindfulness. This is particularly beneficial for seniors, as it helps develop proprioception—the body's ability to sense its position in space. Additionally, this pose can be easily modified to accommodate varying levels of flexibility and strength, making it accessible for all.

Another excellent pose to consider is the Warrior III (Virabhadrasana III), which requires balance, strength, and focus. From a standing position, one leg is lifted behind you while the torso leans forward, creating a straight line from fingertips to toes. This pose engages the core and stabilizing muscles, making it a great choice for athletes looking to refine their balance and body awareness. Furthermore, by practicing Warrior III, you can cultivate mental resilience, as maintaining this pose requires concentration and dedication, qualities that are beneficial in both athletic pursuits and daily life.

Chair Pose (Utkatasana) is also a fantastic option for improving balance while simultaneously building strength in the legs and core. In this pose, individuals squat down as if sitting in an imaginary chair, with arms extended overhead. This position not only challenges balance but also strengthens the lower body, which is vital for overall stability. Practicing Chair Pose regularly can help combat the effects of prolonged sitting, making it particularly useful for office workers and those with sedentary lifestyles. Moreover, this pose promotes mindfulness and body awareness, facilitating a deeper connection between the mind and body.

Lastly, the Half-Moon Pose (Ardha Chandrasana) serves as a powerful balance challenge that enhances flexibility and coordination. From a standing position, one leg is lifted while the opposite hand reaches down to the ground, creating a side stretch. This pose not only improves balance but also encourages the opening of the hips and chest, promoting a sense of lightness and fluidity within the body. Integrating this pose into your routine can be especially beneficial for seniors seeking to maintain mobility and for athletes looking to enhance their agility. Practicing these poses regularly can lead to significant improvements in balance, ultimately contributing to a healthier, more active lifestyle for individuals of all ages.

Integrating Balance Exercises into Daily Life

Integrating balance exercises into daily life is essential for maintaining stability and preventing falls, especially as we age. However, balance is not just a concern for seniors; it is vital for everyone, including parents, office workers, athletes, and youths. By incorporating simple balance exercises into daily routines, individuals can enhance their overall physical health and mental well-being. The key is to embrace these exercises as a natural part of your day rather than viewing them as a chore.

One effective way to integrate balance exercises is by incorporating them into existing activities. For instance, while waiting for water to boil or during commercial breaks while watching television, practice standing on one leg or shifting your weight from one foot to the other. These small adjustments not only improve balance but also help develop core strength and body awareness. Athletes can benefit from this approach by enhancing their stability and coordination, while office workers can counteract the negative effects of prolonged sitting.

Mindfulness plays a crucial role in balance exercises. By focusing on your breath and being present in the moment, you can enhance your connection with your body. This practice encourages a greater awareness of how your body moves and reacts, making it easier to maintain balance. Whether you are a senior practicing restorative yoga or a youth looking to improve athletic performance, mindfulness can enhance the effectiveness of balance exercises, leading to improved mental health and emotional resilience.

Creating a dedicated space for practicing balance exercises can also facilitate their integration into your daily life. Setting aside a specific area in your home or workplace for these practices signals to your mind that it's time to focus on balance and flexibility. This space can be simple, requiring just a mat or a sturdy chair for support. Regularly visiting this space for a few minutes each day can build a habit, ultimately making balance exercises a seamless part of your routine.

Lastly, consider incorporating balance exercises into social activities. Engaging family members or friends in group exercises can make the practice more enjoyable and motivating. Activities like partner yoga or group classes can foster a sense of community and support, making it easier to commit to regular practice. By integrating balance exercises into your daily life in enjoyable and varied ways, you can enhance your stability, improve your physical health, and cultivate mindfulness, benefiting all aspects of life.

Chapter 5: Yoga for Mental Health

Connection Between Yoga and Mental Well-Being

The connection between yoga and mental well-being is a multifaceted relationship that has gained significant attention in recent years. Research continues to demonstrate that yoga can be a powerful tool for enhancing mental health across various demographics, including seniors, office workers, athletes, and youth. The practice encourages mindfulness, fosters relaxation, and promotes emotional balance, making it particularly beneficial for those dealing with stress, anxiety, or depression. Through the integration of breath control, physical postures, and meditation, yoga creates a holistic approach that nurtures both body and mind.

For seniors, engaging in gentle yoga can significantly improve mental well-being by reducing feelings of loneliness and isolation. Many older adults face challenges such as loss of loved ones, physical limitations, and decreased social interactions. Participating in a yoga class offers a supportive community and a shared space for connection. The meditative aspects of yoga also help seniors cultivate mindfulness, allowing them to remain present and engaged in their daily lives, which is essential for mental health. Regular practice promotes a sense of purpose and can mitigate symptoms of anxiety or depression commonly experienced in later life.

Office workers often experience chronic stress due to demanding schedules and work-related pressures. Incorporating yoga into their routines can provide a vital mental health boost, helping to alleviate the negative effects of prolonged sitting and high-stress environments. Simple breathing exercises and stretches can be performed during breaks, leading to increased focus and productivity. Restorative yoga practices, which emphasize relaxation and gentle movements, can also be particularly effective for unwinding after a long day, helping to clear the mind and restore emotional balance.

Athletes, on the other hand, can harness yoga not only for physical flexibility and strength but also for mental resilience. The competitive nature of sports often leads to mental strain, and yoga can serve as a counterbalance. Techniques such as visualization and mindfulness practiced in yoga can enhance concentration and mental clarity, critical components for peak performance. Additionally, yoga fosters an improved mind-body connection, enabling athletes to listen to their bodies better and manage stress and fatigue more effectively, ultimately contributing to their overall mental well-being.

Incorporating yoga into daily life can yield profound benefits for individuals of all ages and backgrounds. Whether one is seeking to alleviate back pain, enhance flexibility and balance, or simply find tranquility amid the chaos of everyday life, yoga offers a versatile approach to mental health. The consistent practice encourages self-awareness and emotional regulation, paving the way for a healthier mindset. As we recognize the importance of mental well-being in our fast-paced world, embracing yoga can be a meaningful step towards achieving greater balance and peace in our lives.

Mindfulness Practices in Yoga

Mindfulness practices in yoga serve as a powerful tool to enhance overall well-being, particularly for seniors, athletes, and anyone seeking a deeper connection to their body and mind. At its core, mindfulness encourages individuals to focus on the present moment, fostering awareness of thoughts, feelings, and physical sensations. This practice is particularly beneficial in yoga, where the combination of breath, movement, and meditation creates a holistic experience that can improve flexibility, balance, and mental clarity. For seniors, incorporating mindfulness into their yoga routine can lead to improved quality of life, reduced stress, and greater physical awareness, making each movement more intentional and beneficial.

One of the key aspects of mindfulness in yoga is the emphasis on breath awareness. Practitioners are encouraged to observe their breathing patterns, noticing the rise and fall of the chest and abdomen. This focus helps ground individuals in the present moment, allowing distractions and worries to fade away. For office workers and busy parents, taking a few minutes to practice mindful breathing can serve as a valuable reset amidst a hectic day. Even simple techniques, such as inhaling for a count of four and exhaling for a count of six, can stimulate relaxation and enhance concentration, making them effective tools for managing stress and anxiety.

Gentle flow yoga classes, designed for seniors and those recovering from injuries, often incorporate mindfulness practices that promote a sense of peace and relaxation. Poses are typically held longer, allowing practitioners to fully engage with each movement and explore their physical limitations and capabilities. This mindful approach not only increases flexibility and strength but also encourages a deeper awareness of one's body, which is crucial for injury prevention. Athletes can benefit from this practice by developing a more profound connection to their physicality, enhancing performance, and reducing the risk of burnout.

Meditation is another essential component of mindfulness in yoga. By integrating brief meditation sessions into a yoga practice, individuals can cultivate a sense of inner calm and clarity. This is especially helpful for seniors who may experience cognitive decline or anxiety. Simple guided meditations focusing on gratitude or body scanning can enhance mental health and emotional resilience. For athletes, meditation can improve focus and mental stamina, providing a competitive edge. It serves as a powerful complement to physical training by allowing them to visualize success and cultivate a positive mindset.

Incorporating mindfulness into daily life extends beyond the mat. Practicing mindfulness during everyday activities, such as eating or walking, can enhance overall awareness and promote a healthier lifestyle. This is particularly important for those looking to manage weight or alleviate back pain. By fostering a mindful approach to movement and nutrition, individuals can make more conscious choices that support their health goals. As mindfulness practices continue to gain recognition within the broader context of yoga, it becomes increasingly clear that the integration of these practices can lead to profound transformations in physical, mental, and emotional well-being for everyone, from seniors to athletes.

Techniques for Stress Relief

Stress relief is a crucial aspect of maintaining overall health and well-being, particularly as we navigate the challenges of daily life. Various techniques can help alleviate stress, and yoga is one of the most effective methods. Practicing yoga promotes relaxation and mindfulness, allowing individuals to connect their body and mind. Through gentle movements and controlled breathing, yoga encourages the release of tension, making it an excellent tool for everyone, including seniors, athletes, and office workers. Incorporating yoga into your routine can foster a sense of calm and resilience in the face of life's pressures.

One powerful technique for stress relief within yoga is mindful breathing. This practice involves focusing on the breath, observing its natural rhythm, and using it as an anchor during moments of anxiety or stress. By concentrating on inhaling and exhaling, individuals can quiet their minds and create a sense of presence. Mindful breathing can be particularly beneficial for seniors and those new to yoga, as it requires minimal physical exertion while providing immediate relaxation. Athletes can also benefit from this technique by using breath control to enhance performance and manage competition-related stress.

Gentle flow sequences in yoga can provide a soothing experience for individuals seeking stress relief. These sequences typically involve slow, deliberate movements that promote flexibility and ease tension in the body. For seniors, gentle flows can improve mobility while reducing stress on joints. Athletes can use these sequences to recover from intense training sessions and prepare their bodies for performance. Engaging in a gentle flow not only nurtures physical well-being but also encourages mental clarity, making it an effective strategy for managing stress.

Restorative yoga is another technique that offers profound stress relief. This form of yoga utilizes props to support the body in restful postures, allowing for deep relaxation and restoration. Restorative yoga is particularly beneficial for individuals experiencing chronic stress or fatigue, as it encourages the nervous system to shift from a state of tension to one of relaxation. For office workers and busy parents, dedicating time to restorative yoga can be a transformative practice, providing a well-deserved break from the demands of daily life.

Incorporating yoga into your daily routine can significantly enhance your stress management toolkit. Combining techniques such as mindful breathing, gentle flow sequences, and restorative practices creates a holistic approach to stress relief. Whether you are a senior looking to improve flexibility, an athlete aiming for balance, or a busy professional seeking calm, the diverse benefits of yoga cater to all demographics. By embracing these techniques, individuals can cultivate resilience, improve mental health, and foster a more balanced lifestyle.

Chapter 6: Restorative Yoga for Seniors

What is Restorative Yoga?

Restorative yoga is a gentle, calming practice that focuses on relaxation and rejuvenation. It is designed to help individuals of all ages and fitness levels, making it particularly beneficial for seniors, office workers, athletes, and anyone looking for a way to unwind and relieve stress. Unlike more vigorous forms of yoga, restorative yoga emphasizes the use of props, such as blankets, bolsters, and straps, to support the body in a variety of poses. This support allows practitioners to hold poses for extended periods, promoting deep relaxation and a sense of peace.

The primary goal of restorative yoga is to activate the body's relaxation response. By encouraging a state of calm, this practice helps to reduce stress and anxiety, making it an excellent choice for those seeking mental clarity and emotional balance. As participants are guided through a series of simple, supported poses, they are encouraged to focus on their breath and the sensations within their bodies. This mindfulness aspect of restorative yoga enhances its effectiveness in promoting overall well-being and mental health, making it suitable for everyone, including busy parents and office workers.

In addition to its mental health benefits, restorative yoga can also support physical health. The gentle stretches and prolonged holds help to improve flexibility, which is particularly important for seniors and athletes aiming to prevent injuries. This practice can aid in alleviating back pain and tension associated with everyday activities or intense training. By fostering greater body awareness, individuals can learn to listen to their bodies and respect their limits, leading to a more mindful approach to movement and exercise.

Restorative yoga can also play a significant role in weight management. Although it may not burn as many calories as more vigorous workouts, the practice encourages a healthier relationship with food and body image. By reducing stress and promoting relaxation, restorative yoga can help combat emotional eating and encourage mindful eating habits. This holistic approach can be particularly valuable for those navigating weight loss journeys, as well as for individuals looking to maintain a balanced lifestyle.

Incorporating restorative yoga into a regular routine can yield profound benefits for people of all ages and backgrounds. Its focus on relaxation and mindfulness can help to create a sense of balance in a fast-paced world, making it an ideal complement to more intense forms of exercise like hot yoga or athletic training. Whether you are a senior seeking gentle movement, a busy professional managing stress, or an athlete looking to enhance recovery, restorative yoga offers a nurturing space to rejuvenate both body and mind.

Benefits of Restorative Practices

Restorative practices, particularly in the context of yoga, offer a multitude of benefits that cater to a diverse audience, including seniors, office workers, athletes, and individuals of all ages. One of the primary advantages of restorative practices is their ability to promote relaxation and reduce stress. In today's fast-paced world, many people experience chronic stress, which can lead to a myriad of health issues, including anxiety, depression, and physical discomfort. Restorative yoga encourages deep relaxation through gentle postures and breathing techniques, allowing practitioners to release tension and cultivate a sense of calm. This state of relaxation is especially beneficial for seniors, who may face heightened stress levels due to various life changes, as well as for office workers dealing with demanding schedules.

Another significant benefit of restorative practices is their capacity to enhance flexibility and balance. Many individuals, particularly seniors and athletes, often struggle with stiffness and decreased mobility. Restorative yoga focuses on gentle stretches and supported poses that promote flexibility without the risk of injury. By holding poses for extended periods, practitioners can gradually increase their range of motion and improve overall body awareness. This is particularly important for seniors, who may experience age-related declines in flexibility, and for athletes looking to recover from intense training while maintaining optimal performance.

Restorative practices also play a vital role in mental health. The integration of mindfulness techniques in restorative yoga encourages individuals to cultivate awareness of their thoughts and feelings without judgment. This practice can be especially beneficial for those dealing with anxiety or depression, as it provides a safe space for self-reflection and emotional release. By fostering a deeper connection between the mind and body, restorative yoga can help individuals develop coping strategies that enhance their overall mental well-being. This aspect is crucial for everyone, from youths navigating the pressures of school to adults managing the complexities of work-life balance.

Furthermore, restorative practices can significantly aid in pain relief and recovery. Many people, including seniors and athletes, often experience chronic pain or discomfort due to various factors such as injuries, posture, or sedentary lifestyles. Restorative yoga utilizes props and supportive postures to alleviate pressure on the body, promoting healing and recovery. Gentle stretching and mindful breathing can help reduce tension in the muscles and improve circulation, making it an effective tool for those suffering from back pain or other physical ailments. This holistic approach to pain management is invaluable for individuals seeking alternatives to medication or invasive treatments.

Finally, restorative practices foster a sense of community and connection among practitioners. Whether in a group class or through shared experiences at home, the practice of restorative yoga encourages individuals to support one another in their journeys toward health and wellness. This sense of belonging is particularly important for seniors and individuals who may feel isolated or disconnected. Engaging in restorative practices together nurtures relationships and creates a supportive environment where participants can share their challenges and successes. Ultimately, the benefits of restorative practices extend beyond the individual, contributing to a healthier, more connected community.

Restorative Poses for Seniors

Restorative poses are an essential component of yoga, particularly beneficial for seniors who may be seeking to enhance their flexibility and balance while also promoting relaxation and mental well-being. These gentle postures focus on rest and recovery, allowing the body to rejuvenate and the mind to unwind. For seniors, restorative yoga can help alleviate tension, reduce stress, and improve overall quality of life, making it an invaluable practice for maintaining health and vitality.

One of the key restorative poses for seniors is the Supported Child's Pose. This pose encourages gentle stretching of the back while providing a sense of security and comfort. By using props such as blankets or bolsters, seniors can modify the pose to suit their needs, allowing for a deeper relaxation experience. This position not only helps to release tension in the spine but also encourages a calming effect on the nervous system, making it particularly beneficial for those dealing with anxiety or stress.

Another valuable pose is the Legs Up the Wall pose, which promotes circulation and helps to relieve swelling in the legs. Seniors can perform this pose by lying on their backs with their legs extended vertically against a wall. This restorative pose encourages relaxation and can provide relief from back pain and discomfort, making it an excellent choice for those who may spend long hours in a seated position. Additionally, this pose aids in calming the mind, offering a moment of mindfulness and tranquility.

The Supported Bridge pose is also an excellent restorative option for seniors, as it strengthens the back, opens the chest, and stretches the front body. By using props like a block or a bolster under the hips, seniors can enjoy the benefits of this pose without straining their bodies. This gentle lift helps alleviate tension in the lower back and encourages deep breathing, further enhancing relaxation and promoting mental clarity. Incorporating this pose into a regular practice can significantly benefit seniors looking to improve their overall well-being.

Lastly, the Savasana, or Corpse Pose, is a fundamental restorative pose that provides an opportunity for deep relaxation and introspection. By lying flat on the back with arms resting comfortably at the sides, seniors can allow their bodies to absorb the benefits of their practice. Savasana encourages mindfulness and mental stillness, making it an ideal pose for relieving stress and promoting emotional balance. Incorporating restorative poses like these into a regular yoga practice can help seniors cultivate a greater sense of peace and well-being, ultimately enhancing their overall quality of life.

Chapter 7: Yoga for Weight Loss

Understanding Weight Management and Yoga

Understanding weight management is a multifaceted endeavor that encompasses physical, mental, and emotional health. For individuals across various demographics, including seniors, athletes, and office workers, integrating yoga into a weight management strategy can provide significant benefits. Yoga promotes physical fitness through movement and flexibility, while also fostering mindfulness and self-awareness, which are essential in maintaining a healthy lifestyle. This holistic approach can empower practitioners to make informed choices about nutrition and exercise, ultimately leading to sustainable weight management.

Yoga can be particularly beneficial for seniors who may face unique challenges related to weight management. As we age, metabolism tends to slow down, and maintaining muscle mass becomes more difficult. Gentle yoga practices enhance flexibility and balance, which are crucial for preventing falls and injuries. Additionally, yoga helps to alleviate stress, a common factor that can lead to emotional eating. By cultivating a mindful approach to eating and movement, seniors can improve their overall well-being and find a more harmonious relationship with their body.

For athletes, weight management is often tied to performance. Yoga complements traditional training regimens by improving flexibility, enhancing breathing techniques, and promoting recovery. The practice encourages athletes to listen to their bodies, which can prevent injuries and promote longevity in their sport. Furthermore, restorative yoga sessions can aid in muscle recovery, allowing athletes to maintain an optimal weight while ensuring their bodies are well-rested and ready for the next challenge.

Office workers, on the other hand, frequently encounter sedentary lifestyles that contribute to weight gain. Incorporating yoga into a daily routine can counteract the effects of prolonged sitting. Simple stretches and mindful breathing exercises can be performed at a desk, helping to reduce stress and tension. This not only promotes physical health but supports mental clarity and productivity. By viewing yoga as a tool for weight management, office workers can create a healthier work environment that fosters both physical and mental well-being.

Lastly, for individuals seeking weight loss or mental health support, yoga provides a unique avenue to explore these goals. The practice encourages self-reflection and emotional regulation, which can be beneficial for those struggling with unhealthy eating patterns. Hot yoga, for instance, can enhance calorie burning through increased heart rates and sweating, while also providing a detoxifying experience. By understanding the various dimensions of weight management through yoga, individuals from all walks of life can discover a path that supports their health goals while promoting a balanced and mindful lifestyle.

Gentle Flow Yoga Sequences for Weight Loss

Gentle flow yoga sequences can be an effective and accessible approach for individuals seeking to lose weight while enhancing flexibility and balance. Unlike more intense forms of exercise, gentle flow yoga emphasizes mindful movement and breath, making it suitable for a diverse audience, including seniors, office workers, parents, and athletes. This practice encourages participants to tune into their bodies, promoting a sense of awareness that can lead to healthier choices both on and off the mat.

In a gentle flow yoga sequence, postures are linked together in a serene manner, allowing for a continuous movement that fosters engagement and focus. This style helps to elevate the heart rate gradually without the risk of injury or excessive strain, making it ideal for those who may be new to exercise or are returning after a long break. By incorporating poses such as sun salutations, lunges, and gentle twists, practitioners enhance their muscle strength and endurance while also supporting weight loss through increased caloric expenditure.

Breath is a fundamental component of any yoga practice, and in gentle flow sequences, it plays a critical role in promoting relaxation and mindfulness. Deep, intentional breathing not only calms the mind but also stimulates the parasympathetic nervous system, which can improve digestion and metabolism. This connection between breath and movement encourages participants to develop a deeper awareness of their bodies, fostering a mindset conducive to making healthier lifestyle choices, including nutrition and physical activity.

In addition to its physical benefits, gentle flow yoga can significantly impact mental health, providing a sanctuary for stress relief and emotional well-being. The gentle nature of the practice allows individuals to cultivate mindfulness, which can help in managing emotional eating and cravings. By learning to be present and attuned to their feelings, practitioners can better understand their relationship with food and develop healthier habits that support their weight loss goals.

Ultimately, gentle flow yoga sequences can be a powerful tool for anyone looking to lose weight while enhancing overall well-being. By integrating gentle movements, mindful breathing, and a focus on mental health, individuals can create a sustainable path toward achieving their fitness goals. Whether you are a busy parent, an office worker, or a senior, these sequences offer a nurturing way to engage with your body, promote weight loss, and foster a sense of balance and flexibility in both mind and body.

Nutrition Tips to Complement Yoga Practice

Nutrition plays a crucial role in enhancing the benefits of yoga practice, particularly for seniors and individuals of varying lifestyles, including athletes and busy office workers. A balanced diet rich in whole foods can provide the necessary energy for yoga sessions while supporting overall health. Incorporating a variety of fruits and vegetables ensures an adequate intake of essential vitamins and minerals, which can help reduce inflammation and improve flexibility. For those engaged in restorative or gentle yoga, focusing on easily digestible foods can enhance relaxation and prevent discomfort during practice.

Hydration is another vital aspect to consider when complementing yoga with proper nutrition. The body loses water through sweat, especially in hot yoga classes, and maintaining hydration is essential for optimal performance and recovery. Drinking water throughout the day, as well as consuming hydrating foods like cucumbers and oranges, can help keep energy levels stable and improve focus during practice. For seniors, staying hydrated aids in maintaining joint health and preventing muscle cramps, which can enhance balance and mobility.

Timing your meals around yoga practice can significantly influence your experience on the mat. Consuming a light snack about an hour before class can provide the necessary energy without feeling overly full. Opt for easily digestible options such as a banana, yogurt, or a small handful of nuts. Post-practice nutrition is equally important; a meal rich in protein and complex carbohydrates can aid recovery and replenish energy stores. Smoothies or bowls with spinach, chia seeds, and berries are excellent choices that support muscle repair while being gentle on the digestive system.

For those practicing yoga for weight loss or mental health, focusing on mindful eating can amplify the benefits of yoga. Being aware of hunger cues and eating slowly can foster a healthier relationship with food, making it easier to choose nourishing options. Incorporating mindfulness techniques learned in yoga can assist in making conscious food choices, ultimately supporting weight management and emotional well-being. This approach not only complements the physical aspects of yoga but also enhances mental clarity and reduces stress.

Lastly, tailored nutrition strategies are beneficial for specific practices within yoga. Athletes may benefit from higher protein intake to support muscle recovery, while seniors might focus on nutrient-dense foods that promote bone health, such as leafy greens and fortified dairy products. For individuals dealing with back pain or seeking mindfulness, incorporating anti-inflammatory foods like turmeric and fatty fish can provide additional support. By aligning nutrition with yoga goals, practitioners can cultivate a holistic approach to well-being that fosters flexibility, balance, and overall health.

Chapter 8: Yoga for Back Pain Relief

Common Causes of Back Pain in Seniors

Back pain is a prevalent issue among seniors, often stemming from a combination of age-related changes in the body and various lifestyle factors. One of the most common causes is the natural degeneration of the spine and its components. As individuals age, the intervertebral discs, which act as cushions between the vertebrae, lose hydration and elasticity, leading to a reduction in their effectiveness. This can result in conditions such as osteoarthritis or degenerative disc disease, which contribute to discomfort and limited mobility.

Another significant contributor to back pain in seniors is muscle weakness and loss of flexibility. As people age, they tend to become less active, leading to a decline in muscle strength and flexibility. This reduction can create an imbalance in the musculoskeletal system, making it more susceptible to strains and injuries. Weak core muscles, specifically, can fail to provide adequate support for the spine, exacerbating back pain. Engaging in gentle yoga practices can help strengthen these muscles, promoting better posture and alignment.

Postural issues are also a common cause of back pain among older adults. Many seniors develop poor posture due to prolonged periods of sitting, often from sedentary lifestyles or extended hours at desks. This can lead to misalignment of the spine and increased strain on the back muscles. Activities that encourage mindfulness and proper body mechanics, such as yoga, can help seniors become more aware of their posture and make necessary adjustments to reduce pain and discomfort.

Chronic conditions and previous injuries can further complicate the experience of back pain in seniors. Conditions such as arthritis, osteoporosis, or previous spinal injuries may predispose older adults to recurrent discomfort. Additionally, the psychological aspect of living with chronic pain can lead to increased tension and stress, which may manifest physically as muscle tightness. Incorporating restorative yoga and mindfulness into daily routines can aid in alleviating not only physical pain but also the mental toll associated with chronic conditions.

In conclusion, understanding the common causes of back pain in seniors is crucial for developing effective management strategies. Identifying factors such as spinal degeneration, muscle weakness, postural issues, and chronic conditions can guide seniors in making informed decisions about their health. Gentle yoga practices, with a focus on enhancing flexibility, strength, and mindfulness, can be an invaluable tool in alleviating back pain and improving overall quality of life. By integrating these practices into their daily routines, seniors can take proactive steps towards maintaining their physical and mental well-being.

Effective Yoga Poses for Relief

Incorporating yoga into daily routines can offer a multitude of benefits, particularly for those seeking relief from physical discomfort or mental stress. This section focuses on specific yoga poses that are gentle yet effective, catering to a broad audience ranging from seniors to busy office workers and athletes. Each pose is designed to enhance flexibility, improve balance, and provide therapeutic relief for common ailments such as back pain, stress, and anxiety.

One of the most accessible poses for everyone is the Cat-Cow stretch. This dynamic movement not only warms up the spine but also promotes flexibility and releases tension in the back. Starting on all fours, participants alternate between arching their back and rounding it, synchronized with their breath. This gentle flow helps to ease stiffness and improve overall spinal health, making it particularly beneficial for seniors and those who spend long hours sitting at desks.

Another effective pose is the Child's Pose, which is known for its restorative properties. This pose encourages deep relaxation and is excellent for relieving tension in the back, neck, and shoulders. By kneeling and resting the forehead on the mat, individuals can focus on their breath, promoting mindfulness while gently stretching the hips and thighs. This pose is suitable for all ages and fitness levels, making it a versatile option for anyone looking to alleviate stress and find tranquility.

For individuals dealing with back pain, the Supported Bridge Pose offers significant relief. By lying on the back with knees bent and feet flat on the floor, participants can lift their hips while supporting their lower back with a cushion or block. This pose not only strengthens the back and glutes but also opens the chest, allowing for deeper breathing. Incorporating this pose into a routine can help alleviate discomfort and promote better posture, which is essential for both seniors and athletes.

Finally, the Legs-Up-the-Wall pose serves as an excellent restorative option for improving circulation and calming the nervous system. By lying on their backs with legs extended up against a wall, individuals can experience a gentle inversion that promotes relaxation and reduces swelling in the legs. This pose is particularly beneficial for office workers who may experience fatigue from prolonged sitting, as well as seniors looking to enhance circulation. By integrating these effective yoga poses into their lives, individuals can find relief from both physical and mental stress, fostering a greater sense of well-being.

Creating a Back Pain Relief Routine

Back pain is a common issue that can affect individuals of all ages and lifestyles, from office workers hunched over desks to athletes pushing their physical limits. Establishing a consistent back pain relief routine can make a significant difference in managing discomfort and enhancing overall well-being. This routine should include a combination of gentle yoga stretches, strengthening exercises, and mindfulness practices tailored to individual needs and capabilities.

The foundation of an effective back pain relief routine lies in gentle yoga poses that promote flexibility and strength in the back muscles. Poses such as Cat-Cow, Child's Pose, and Downward-Facing Dog can help alleviate tension and improve spinal alignment. These poses encourage movement and stretching of the back, gradually reducing stiffness and promoting greater range of motion. For seniors or those with limited mobility, modifications can be made to ensure safety and comfort while still reaping the benefits of these foundational stretches.

In addition to stretching, strengthening the core muscles is essential for providing support to the spine and preventing future back pain. Incorporating poses like Bridge and Plank can strengthen the abdominal and lower back muscles. It is important to focus on maintaining proper alignment and engaging the core throughout these exercises to avoid strain. For individuals who may find it challenging to perform these poses on the floor, seated variations can be introduced to accommodate their needs.

Mindfulness and breathwork are integral components of a back pain relief routine. Incorporating deep breathing techniques, such as diaphragmatic breathing, can help release tension in the body and promote relaxation. Practicing mindfulness during yoga sessions encourages individuals to connect with their bodies, recognize pain signals, and respond with compassion. This awareness can lead to better management of pain and a deeper understanding of how emotional stress may contribute to physical discomfort.

Finally, consistency is key in any back pain relief routine. Setting aside dedicated time each day or several times a week to practice yoga can lead to significant improvements over time. Keeping a journal to track progress and reflect on changes in pain levels can also be beneficial. By combining gentle stretches, strengthening exercises, and mindfulness techniques, individuals can create a comprehensive routine that not only addresses back pain but also enhances overall physical and mental health.

Chapter 9: Yoga and Mindfulness

The Role of Mindfulness in Yoga

The practice of mindfulness is integral to yoga, serving as a bridge that connects physical movement with mental clarity. Mindfulness in yoga encourages practitioners to become fully aware of their breath, body, and thoughts, fostering an environment where they can observe their experiences without judgment. For seniors, this awareness can lead to improved balance and flexibility, as they learn to listen to their bodies and respond to its needs. Mindfulness helps reduce the risk of injury by promoting careful, intentional movements, allowing seniors to engage in yoga safely and effectively.

For athletes, mindfulness enhances performance by sharpening focus and concentration. By incorporating mindfulness into their yoga practice, athletes can develop a deeper awareness of their body mechanics and mental states, leading to improved technique and reduced mental fatigue. This heightened awareness can translate into better performance in their respective sports, as athletes learn to manage stress and stay present during competition. Moreover, mindfulness helps athletes recover more effectively by promoting relaxation and reducing tension, which is essential for maintaining peak physical condition.

In the realm of mental health, mindfulness serves as a powerful tool for stress reduction and emotional regulation. Practicing yoga with a focus on mindfulness enables individuals to cultivate a sense of peace and stability, even amidst life's challenges. This practice can be particularly beneficial for seniors who may face various life transitions, providing them with a sense of purpose and connection. Restorative yoga, combined with mindfulness, can help alleviate symptoms of anxiety and depression, offering a gentle way to promote mental well-being.

Weight loss efforts can also benefit from the integration of mindfulness into yoga practice. By encouraging mindfulness, individuals become more attuned to their hunger cues and emotional triggers, fostering healthier eating habits. This heightened awareness can lead to more conscious choices regarding nutrition and exercise, enhancing overall wellness. Mindful yoga practices promote a positive relationship with food and body image, allowing practitioners to approach weight loss with compassion rather than restriction.

Lastly, mindfulness plays a crucial role in addressing specific physical concerns, such as back pain relief. By focusing on breath and body awareness, practitioners can identify areas of tension and discomfort, leading to more effective management of pain. Gentle flow yoga encourages slow, mindful movements that promote healing and flexibility in the spine. Through mindfulness, individuals learn to cultivate patience and resilience, essential qualities that support both physical and emotional healing. This holistic approach makes yoga a valuable practice for seniors and individuals of all ages seeking to enhance their overall quality of life.

Techniques to Cultivate Mindfulness

Cultivating mindfulness is an essential practice that can enhance overall well-being, regardless of age or lifestyle. Mindfulness involves being fully present in the moment, acknowledging thoughts and feelings without judgment. For seniors, incorporating mindfulness into daily routines can help reduce stress and improve mental clarity. Athletes can benefit from mindfulness to enhance focus and performance, while office workers may find it aids in managing work-related stress. By integrating mindfulness into yoga practices, individuals can develop a deeper connection to their bodies and minds, fostering a sense of balance and peace.

One effective technique to cultivate mindfulness is through breath awareness. Focusing on the breath allows individuals to anchor themselves in the present moment. In yoga, this can be practiced by taking slow, deep breaths, inhaling through the nose and exhaling through the mouth. This technique can be particularly beneficial for seniors and those with back pain, as it encourages relaxation and eases tension in the body. Athletes can also use breath awareness to improve performance, as it helps in regulating energy levels and maintaining composure during competitions.

Another valuable technique is body scanning, where individuals mentally check in with different parts of their bodies. This practice encourages awareness of physical sensations and can be particularly useful for those recovering from injuries or managing chronic pain. During a yoga session, participants can lie down comfortably, close their eyes, and systematically focus on each area of the body, from the toes to the head. By acknowledging feelings of tension or discomfort without judgment, practitioners can foster a greater sense of body awareness and acceptance.

Mindful movement is yet another technique that can be seamlessly integrated into yoga practices. This involves moving through postures with deliberate attention to how each movement feels in the body. For seniors, gentle movements can help in enhancing flexibility and balance, while athletes can improve their physical performance through this increased awareness. Practicing mindful movement allows individuals to cultivate a deeper connection between mind and body, fostering a sense of calm and focus that can carry into daily activities.

Lastly, incorporating gratitude into mindfulness practices can significantly enhance emotional well-being. Taking a moment during or after a yoga session to reflect on what one is grateful for can shift focus from stress and negativity to positivity and appreciation. This technique can be particularly empowering for office workers and individuals managing mental health challenges, as it promotes a more optimistic outlook. By regularly practicing gratitude, individuals of all ages can cultivate a greater sense of mindfulness, leading to improved mental health and overall quality of life.

Daily Mindfulness Practices

Daily mindfulness practices serve as a foundational element for enhancing mental well-being and physical health. Incorporating mindfulness into your daily routine can benefit a diverse range of individuals, from seniors seeking to improve their balance and flexibility to office workers aiming to reduce stress and enhance productivity. Mindfulness involves being present in the moment, cultivating awareness of your thoughts, feelings, and bodily sensations without judgment. This practice can lead to improved focus, emotional regulation, and overall quality of life.

For seniors, daily mindfulness practices can be particularly beneficial. Engaging in gentle yoga and mindful breathing exercises can help alleviate anxiety and promote relaxation. Simple acts, such as focusing on your breath while seated in a comfortable chair, can create a calming effect and enhance your sense of presence. Additionally, integrating mindfulness into daily activities—like mindful walking or enjoying a meal without distractions—can help seniors connect more deeply with their environment and experiences, thereby enhancing mental clarity and emotional resilience.

Athletes, on the other hand, can utilize mindfulness to improve performance and recovery. Mindfulness practices, such as visualization techniques and body scans, can enhance focus and reduce pre-competition anxiety. By training the mind to remain present and aware, athletes can better manage stress, improve their concentration, and cultivate a greater sense of control over their physical and mental states. This heightened awareness can also facilitate a more profound connection with their bodies, allowing for more effective recovery and injury prevention.

For individuals seeking mental health benefits, incorporating mindfulness into daily routines can serve as a powerful tool for managing stress and improving emotional well-being. Mindfulness meditation, which can be practiced for just a few minutes each day, encourages a non-judgmental observation of thoughts and feelings. This practice allows individuals to develop a greater understanding of their mental patterns, helping them navigate challenges with greater ease. Furthermore, restorative yoga sessions that emphasize mindfulness can offer a nurturing space for individuals to reconnect with themselves and foster self-compassion.

Regardless of your background or lifestyle, there are myriad ways to integrate mindfulness into your daily life. Simple practices, such as mindful stretching during yoga sessions, taking a few moments to focus on your breath before starting the day, or practicing gratitude through journaling, can all enhance your mindfulness journey. By dedicating even a small portion of your day to mindfulness, you can cultivate a greater sense of balance, flexibility, and overall well-being, making it an essential complement to your yoga practice and daily life.

Chapter 10: Exploring Hot Yoga

What is Hot Yoga?

Hot yoga is a form of yoga practiced in a heated room, typically set to temperatures around 90 to 105 degrees Fahrenheit. This unique environment is designed to facilitate a deeper stretch and increased flexibility, making it particularly appealing to various demographics, including seniors, athletes, and those looking to enhance their overall wellness. The warmth encourages muscle relaxation, allowing participants to safely deepen their poses and improve their range of motion. This is especially beneficial for seniors who may face challenges with traditional yoga practices due to stiffness or limited mobility.

The practice of hot yoga usually involves a series of postures that focus on strength, balance, and flexibility. While many associate hot yoga with intense workouts, it can be adapted to suit different fitness levels. For seniors, modifications can be made to ensure safety and comfort while still reaping the benefits of the practice. The heat not only helps to warm the muscles but also promotes detoxification through sweating, which can enhance the overall effectiveness of each session. This aspect of hot yoga is particularly appealing to those looking to lose weight or improve their physical fitness.

In addition to the physical benefits, hot yoga can have a positive impact on mental health. The heated environment encourages mindfulness, allowing practitioners to focus on their breath and body sensations without distractions. This meditative aspect can be particularly helpful for busy office workers or parents who often juggle multiple responsibilities. By dedicating time to practice in a hot yoga setting, individuals can cultivate a sense of calm and reduce stress, ultimately enhancing their mental clarity and emotional well-being.

Ultimately, hot yoga offers a versatile approach to fitness and wellness that can benefit a wide range of individuals. Whether you are a senior looking to improve flexibility, an athlete aiming for better performance, or someone seeking mental clarity and stress relief, hot yoga can be tailored to meet your unique needs. By embracing the warmth of the practice, participants can enjoy the physical and mental benefits that come with it, making it an essential component of a holistic approach to health and wellness.

Benefits and Risks for Seniors

The practice of yoga offers numerous benefits for seniors, particularly in enhancing flexibility and balance, which are crucial as individuals age. One of the primary advantages is the improvement in mobility. Many seniors experience stiffness and reduced range of motion, which can hinder daily activities. Through gentle flow yoga, seniors can engage in poses that stretch and strengthen muscles, leading to greater ease in movement. Enhanced flexibility also contributes to better posture, reducing the risk of falls and injuries, which are common concerns for older adults.

In addition to physical benefits, yoga plays a significant role in promoting mental health among seniors. The practice encourages mindfulness and relaxation, which can help alleviate symptoms of anxiety and depression. As seniors often face various life transitions, including retirement or the loss of loved ones, establishing a regular yoga routine can provide a sense of stability and purpose. The meditative aspects of yoga foster a greater sense of awareness and presence, allowing seniors to cultivate peace of mind and emotional well-being.

However, it is essential to acknowledge the risks associated with yoga for seniors. Certain poses may pose challenges, particularly for those with pre-existing conditions or limited mobility. This makes it crucial for seniors to consult with healthcare providers before starting a yoga practice. Modifications may be necessary to ensure safety and comfort. Classes specifically designed for seniors, led by qualified instructors, can help mitigate these risks by providing tailored instructions and adjustments that cater to individual abilities.

Another notable risk is the potential for overexertion. Seniors may feel motivated to push their limits, especially when they see improvements in their flexibility and strength. It is important for participants to listen to their bodies and recognize when to rest. Striving for progress should not come at the expense of safety, and seniors must be mindful of their physical limits. Incorporating restorative yoga practices can be beneficial, as they focus on gentle movements and relaxation, allowing for recovery while still promoting overall health.

Ultimately, the benefits of yoga for seniors often outweigh the risks when approached mindfully. By enhancing flexibility, balance, and mental well-being, yoga can significantly improve quality of life. Seniors who adopt a gentle flow yoga practice can experience physical rejuvenation and emotional resilience. With the right precautions and guidance, they can enjoy the myriad benefits while minimizing potential dangers, making yoga a valuable addition to their wellness routine.

Modifications for Safe Practice

Modifications for safe practice in yoga are essential for ensuring that practitioners of all ages and abilities can participate without risk of injury. As individuals engage in yoga, particularly seniors, athletes, or those with specific physical concerns, understanding how to adapt poses to suit their personal needs is crucial. This individualized approach not only enhances the physical benefits of yoga but also supports mental health by fostering a sense of empowerment and confidence in one's practice.

One of the primary modifications involves the use of props such as blocks, straps, and bolsters. These tools can help practitioners achieve proper alignment and deepen their stretches without straining. For seniors or those with mobility issues, blocks can be placed under the hands during standing poses to reduce the distance to the floor. Straps can assist in reaching for the feet in seated stretches, ensuring that the practitioner maintains a safe range of motion.

Another important aspect of modifications is the adjustment of posture intensity. Practitioners should **listen to their bodies** and avoid pushing into pain. For instance, in forward bends, it may be more beneficial to keep the knees slightly bent rather than forcing the stretch. This modification can be particularly useful for individuals with back pain or tight hamstrings. Additionally, restorative yoga poses can be introduced to promote relaxation and recovery, especially for those experiencing stress or fatigue from intense training or daily life.

Incorporating chair yoga is also a valuable modification for those who may struggle with traditional floor-based poses. This practice allows seniors and individuals with limited mobility to experience the benefits of yoga while remaining seated. It provides a safe way to enhance flexibility and balance without the risk of falling or overexertion. Chair yoga can be particularly appealing to office workers who may spend long hours sitting, seniors or anyone with limited mobility as it offers a way to stretch and move without needing extensive space or equipment.

Finally, mindfulness plays a critical role in safe yoga practice. Encouraging practitioners to focus on their breath and body sensations helps cultivate an awareness that can guide them in making appropriate modifications. This mindfulness approach can significantly reduce the likelihood of injury, as individuals become more attuned to their limits and capabilities. By fostering a gentle and compassionate yoga practice, everyone—regardless of age or fitness level—can experience the transformative benefits of yoga while maintaining safety and well-being.

Chapter 11: Integrating Yoga into Daily Life

Creating a Personal Yoga Routine

Creating a personal yoga routine is an essential step in cultivating a practice that caters specifically to your individual needs and goals. Whether you are a senior looking to enhance flexibility and balance, an athlete aiming to improve performance, or someone seeking mental health benefits through restorative yoga, tailoring your routine can significantly enhance your experience. Start by assessing your current physical condition, flexibility, and any specific areas of concern, such as back pain or weight loss goals. Understanding your body's limitations and strengths will help you select poses and sequences that are both beneficial and safe.

When designing your routine, consider the duration and frequency that fits your lifestyle. Some short, focused sessions that can be done in 15 to 30 minutes might be most beneficial. Conversely, if you have more time, longer sessions can incorporate a wider variety of poses and mindfulness practices. Aim to practice at least three times a week to establish a consistent habit. Be sure to include a mix of gentle stretching and strengthening poses that promote balance, flexibility, and relaxation.

Incorporating mindfulness into your yoga routine is vital for enhancing mental health and overall well-being. Start each session with a few moments of breath awareness, allowing yourself to connect with your intentions for the practice. You may choose to meditate briefly on your goals—whether they are to relieve stress, improve physical health, or cultivate a deeper sense of peace. Mindfulness can be woven throughout your practice by focusing on the sensations in your body, observing your breath, and maintaining a non-judgmental attitude toward your progress. This approach not only enriches the physical benefits of yoga but also promotes emotional resilience.

As you become more familiar with various poses, consider incorporating specific sequences that address your individual needs. For seniors, gentle flows focusing on stability and balance are crucial. Athletes may benefit from dynamic sequences that build strength and improve flexibility in key muscle groups. Additionally, restorative poses can be included for those looking to alleviate stress, while specific stretches can target areas of tension, such as the back. Tailoring your routine in this manner ensures that it serves your unique objectives, whether those are physical, emotional, or a combination of both.

Finally, remember that your yoga routine should be a reflection of your journey. It is essential to remain open to adjusting your practice as your body changes over time. Listening to your body and honoring its signals will help prevent injury and enhance overall enjoyment. Consider keeping a journal to track your progress, noting how you feel before and after each session. This reflection will aid in recognizing patterns and refining your routine further, allowing you to create a deeply personal and effective practice that supports your health and wellness goals.

Tips for Staying Motivated

Staying motivated in any practice, including yoga, can be challenging, especially for seniors or individuals with busy lifestyles. One effective tip to maintain motivation is to establish a consistent schedule. By committing to specific days and times for your yoga practice, you create a routine that becomes part of your daily life. This consistency helps to reinforce the habit, making it easier to integrate yoga into your lifestyle. Consider setting reminders on your phone or using a calendar to keep track of your sessions, whether they are restorative yoga classes or more vigorous practices aimed at building strength and flexibility.

Another way to stay motivated is to set realistic and achievable goals. Whether you're aiming to enhance flexibility, relieve back pain, or improve mental health, defining clear objectives can provide a sense of purpose. Start with small milestones, such as mastering a particular pose or dedicating a few minutes each day to mindfulness during your practice. Celebrate these achievements, no matter how minor they may seem, as they contribute to your overall progress. This approach not only boosts your confidence but also keeps you engaged in your yoga journey.

Incorporating variety into your practice is essential to maintain enthusiasm. Explore different styles of yoga, such as hot yoga or restorative yoga, to keep things fresh and exciting. Each style offers unique benefits, catering to various needs, whether it's enhancing athletic performance, promoting relaxation, or supporting weight loss. By diversifying your sessions, you can prevent boredom and discover new aspects of yoga that resonate with you. Additionally, attending workshops or classes with different instructors can infuse new energy into your routine and provide fresh insights into your practice.

Connecting with a community can also significantly enhance your motivation. Engaging with fellow yoga practitioners, whether in person or online, fosters a sense of belonging and accountability. Many studios offer classes tailored for seniors, athletes, or individuals seeking mental health support, allowing you to meet others with similar goals. Sharing experiences, challenges, and successes with others can inspire you to stay committed and push through difficult days. Consider joining a local yoga group or participating in online forums where you can exchange tips, resources, and encouragement.

Finally, remember to cultivate a positive mindset towards your yoga journey. It's essential to practice self-compassion and recognize that each person's journey is unique. There may be days when motivation wanes or when physical limitations pose challenges. Instead of focusing on perfection, embrace progress and the joy of practicing yoga. Incorporate mindfulness techniques to stay present and acknowledge your feelings without judgment. This approach can reinforce your connection to yoga and help you maintain motivation through both the highs and lows of your practice.

Community Resources and Support

Community resources and support play a crucial role in enhancing the practice of yoga, especially for seniors seeking to improve flexibility and balance. Local community centers often host classes specifically tailored for older adults, providing a welcoming environment where participants can learn and practice yoga with their peers. These classes not only focus on gentle movements but also foster social connections, which can significantly contribute to mental well-being. Engaging in group settings allows seniors to share experiences, encourage one another, and create a sense of belonging that can enhance motivation and consistency in their practice.

In addition to community centers, many gyms and fitness studios offer specialized yoga programs for various demographics, including athletes and office workers. These programs often integrate techniques that address specific needs, such as improving flexibility for athletes or relieving tension for those who spend long hours at a desk. By tapping into these resources, individuals can find classes designed to meet their unique requirements, ensuring that their yoga practice is both effective and enjoyable. The availability of diverse classes also means that everyone, regardless of age or fitness level, can benefit from the restorative properties of yoga.

Online platforms have expanded access to yoga resources, providing an abundance of classes and tutorials that cater to different interests and needs. For those interested in mental health, many reputable yoga instructors offer sessions focused on mindfulness and stress relief. This virtual approach allows participants to practice in the comfort of their own homes, making it more convenient to integrate yoga into daily routines. Furthermore, online communities often host discussions and support groups, creating a space for individuals to share their journeys and learn from one another.

Support from healthcare professionals can also enhance a yoga practice, especially for seniors and those dealing with chronic pain or other health conditions. Many physical therapists and wellness coaches recognize the benefits of yoga and may recommend specific practices to aid in recovery and rehabilitation. Collaborating with healthcare providers ensures that individuals are practicing safely and effectively, addressing any underlying issues while enjoying the benefits of yoga. This integration of yoga into a holistic health plan empowers participants to take charge of their well-being.

Finally, local and online workshops, retreats, and seminars offer additional opportunities for individuals to deepen their understanding of yoga and its benefits. These events often feature experienced instructors who provide personalized guidance, allowing participants to explore various aspects of yoga, including restorative techniques and approaches to weight loss. By investing time in these resources, individuals can cultivate a more profound connection to their practice, ultimately enhancing their physical and mental health. Community support and resources are essential for fostering a sustainable yoga journey that benefits everyone, from seniors to athletes, and promotes overall well-being.

Chapter 12: Conclusion and Next Steps

Reflecting on Your Yoga Journey

Reflecting on your yoga journey can be a transformative experience, allowing individuals from all walks of life to assess their progress, challenges, and personal growth. For seniors, incorporating gentle yoga practices can significantly enhance flexibility and balance, leading to improved mobility and quality of life. As you consider your journey, think about how the principles of yoga have influenced not only your physical capabilities but also your mental and emotional well-being. Each session on the mat can serve as a reminder of the resilience and strength that resides within you, nurturing a deeper connection to your body and mind.

For office workers and athletes, yoga offers a unique opportunity to counteract the physical strains associated with prolonged sitting or intense training. Reflecting on how yoga has complemented your daily routine can illuminate the ways it helps alleviate tension, improve focus, and enhance performance. Whether it's through restorative poses that relieve back pain or dynamic flows that build strength, acknowledging these benefits can motivate you to continue prioritizing yoga as an essential element of your health regimen. The mindful practice encourages you to listen to your body's needs, fostering a sense of self-awareness that can lead to more effective training and recovery.

The mental health benefits of yoga are profound and often overlooked in traditional fitness discussions. Many people, including youth and women, find that yoga serves as a sanctuary where they can explore and manage their emotions. Reflecting on your experiences can reveal how yoga has provided a safe space for stress relief and emotional processing. Whether through mindfulness techniques or intentional breathing exercises, the practice encourages you to cultivate a calm mind and a balanced emotional state. This reflective practice can lead to a deeper understanding of your mental health journey and the role yoga plays in maintaining it.

As you consider your weight loss journey, it's essential to recognize that yoga is not just about physical transformation but holistic well-being. Reflecting on the changes you've experienced can help you appreciate the relationship between body, mind, and spirit. By embracing a gentle flow, you might find that the focus shifts from merely losing weight to fostering a healthy lifestyle that honors your body's needs. This perspective can empower you to make sustainable choices that support your overall health and well-being, rather than engaging in quick-fix diets or intense workout regimens that may not serve you in the long run.

Finally, reflecting on your yoga journey can serve as a powerful tool for personal growth and self-discovery. Each practice, whether in a hot yoga class or a peaceful restorative session, contributes to your evolving understanding of flexibility, balance, and mindfulness. As you continue to engage with yoga, take the time to evaluate how far you've come and where you wish to go. This reflection can inspire you to set new intentions, deepen your practice, and embrace the journey ahead with an open heart and mind. By recognizing the cumulative benefits of yoga, you can cultivate a more meaningful and enriching relationship with your practice, regardless of your age or lifestyle.

Setting Future Goals

Setting future goals is an essential aspect of any yoga practice, particularly for seniors and individuals looking to enhance flexibility and balance. Goal-setting helps create a clear path for personal development, enabling practitioners to focus their efforts on specific outcomes. Whether you are a senior hoping to improve your mobility, an athlete aiming to increase performance, or someone seeking mental clarity through restorative yoga, establishing measurable and attainable goals is crucial for progress. By understanding the importance of these goals, you can tailor your practice to align with your individual needs and aspirations.

When setting future goals, it is important to consider both short-term and long-term objectives. Short-term goals may include mastering a specific yoga pose or improving your range of motion over the next few weeks. These smaller, achievable targets can provide motivation and a sense of accomplishment as you progress in your practice. Long-term goals, on the other hand, might involve developing a consistent yoga routine that supports overall health, aids in weight loss, or alleviates back pain over several months or years. By breaking down larger aspirations into manageable steps, you create a roadmap that guides your practice while allowing for adjustments along the way.

In addition to physical goals, it is vital to incorporate mental and emotional objectives into your yoga journey. Many practitioners find that yoga enhances mindfulness, reduces stress, and fosters a sense of inner peace. Setting goals related to mental health can include committing to daily meditation, practicing gratitude, or participating in yoga classes focused on restorative techniques. These psychological benefits are essential to a holistic approach to well-being, allowing you to cultivate resilience and balance in your life.

As you set your future goals, remember to stay flexible and open to change. Life circumstances may alter your aspirations or the methods you use to achieve them. Embracing this adaptability is crucial, especially for seniors or those with varying physical abilities. Consider seeking guidance from experienced instructors who can help you modify poses and practices to meet your evolving needs. Engaging with a supportive community can also enhance your motivation and accountability, making it easier to stay committed to your goals.

Finally, it is essential to regularly evaluate your progress and celebrate your achievements, no matter how small. Reflecting on your journey can provide valuable insights into what works for you and what areas may require adjustment. By acknowledging your growth, you reinforce positive habits and strengthen your commitment to your yoga practice. Whether you are an office worker seeking relief from stress, an athlete looking to enhance performance, or a senior focusing on flexibility, setting future goals is a powerful tool to enhance your yoga experience and overall quality of life.

Resources for Continued Learning

In the journey of practicing yoga, especially for seniors, continued learning is essential to enhance flexibility, balance, and overall well-being. Various resources are available to support individuals of all ages and backgrounds in their yoga practice. Books, online courses, workshops, and local classes can provide valuable insights and techniques to deepen your understanding of yoga. Engaging with diverse resources keeps the practice fresh and allows practitioners to discover new aspects of yoga that can be tailored to their unique needs.

Books specifically focused on yoga for seniors can offer guidance on modifying poses and incorporating restorative practices. Many authors share their expertise in adapting yoga to enhance physical and mental health, addressing common issues such as back pain, balance challenges, and flexibility limitations. Titles that focus on gentle flow sequences often include illustrations and step-by-step instructions, making them accessible for practitioners at any level. Additionally, books on mindfulness and mental health can complement yoga practice, helping individuals develop a deeper connection to their breath and body.

Online platforms have revolutionized how practitioners access yoga instruction. Websites and apps dedicated to yoga offer a wealth of videos and tutorials that cater to various skill levels and specific needs. Many instructors provide classes focusing on gentle yoga, restorative practices, or targeted sessions for athletes looking to improve their performance and recovery. These resources can be particularly beneficial for those who may prefer practicing at home, allowing them to explore different styles and find what resonates best with their body and mind.

Workshops and local classes are another excellent way to continue learning about yoga. Many studios offer specialized classes for seniors, athletes, or those seeking to address specific health concerns. Attending workshops led by experienced instructors can provide hands-on adjustments and personalized feedback, enhancing the overall experience. Additionally, community centers and fitness facilities often host seminars on topics related to yoga and mindfulness, providing opportunities for practitioners to engage with experts and fellow yoga enthusiasts.

Finally, engaging with online forums and social media groups can foster a sense of community among yoga practitioners. These platforms allow individuals to share their experiences, ask questions, and exchange tips on maintaining a consistent yoga practice. By connecting with others, practitioners can gain motivation and inspiration while learning from the diverse experiences of their peers. As the practice evolves, these resources will encourage continued growth and exploration, ultimately enhancing the benefits of yoga for seniors and individuals at any stage of life.